Aging Reverse Mastery

Step 1: How to Stay Fit with 1 Hour a Day of Movement

ESTHER KING

Legal & Disclaimer

Legal & Disclaimer

The information contained in this book is not designed to replace or take the place of any form of medicine or professional medical advice. The information in this book has been provided for educational and entertainment purposes only.

The information contained in this book has been compiled from sources deemed reliable, and it is accurate to the best of the Author's knowledge; however, the Author cannot guarantee its accuracy and validity and cannot be held liable for any errors or omissions. Changes are periodically made to this book. You must consult your doctor or get professional medical advice before using any of the suggested remedies, techniques, or information in this book.

Upon using the information contained in this book, you agree to hold harmless the Author from and against any damages, costs, and expenses, including any legal fees potentially resulting from the application of any of the information provided by this guide. This disclaimer applies to any damages or injury caused by the use and application, whether directly or indirectly, of any advice or information presented, whether for breach of contract, tort, negligence, personal injury, criminal intent, or under any other cause of action.

Table of Contents

Introduction

Aging. It's one of those things that we all don't like to admit it, but we do really fear the process. We worry about what our bodies are going to look like, how we are going to feel, and whether or not we will be able to keep up with the rest of our families.

You don't have to be afraid of aging, however, if you do some preventative maintenance to keep yourself in good physical shape. This doesn't mean that you have to weigh 120 pounds and run twelve miles every day. That isn't what you need. Instead, we will go back to something that you learned in high school, and that is Newton's First Law of Motion:

> An object at rest stays at rest and an object in motion stays in motion with the same speed and in the same direction unless acted upon by an unbalanced force.

You want to be that object that stays in motion. Simply getting up and walking to the mailbox every day or walking around your local grocery store isn't enough to stop the aging process.

Think about how you used to move: you ran after your children, you walked all day at work, you walked the dog, and you likely just walked more in your day to day activities. Now that you started slowing down and doing less? It is going to be harder and harder to find the energy to keep it up.

This book isn't meant to scare you into joining the gym. Instead, it is to keep you moving! You will learn different ways to stay moving so that you can feel better and participate in daily activities.

You can pick and choose which of these activities feel best for you and which ones will work with your lifestyle. It's up to you to change your future and make yourself feel better.

We start with you giving yourself just one hour a day – one hour where you selfishly work on yourself and no one else.

What is Aging Anyway?

Aging. It is something you hear about and many of us will treat it like a four letter word. It is something that is inevitable: our hair will turn gray, our skin will lose elasticity, we won't be able to lift as much, our bones will weaken, and we will slow down.

You cannot stop aging, so you might as well learn to work with it.

In the broadest sense of the word, aging encompasses all of the changes that you will go through over a lifetime. You develop, you grow, you reach maturity – all from the day you were born.

To those who are young, aging means exciting opportunities – you can go to the movies alone, you can drive a car, you can vote, you can drink, and many even celebrate when they reach the age of social security. But one day that all stops and you aren't looking forward to aging anymore.

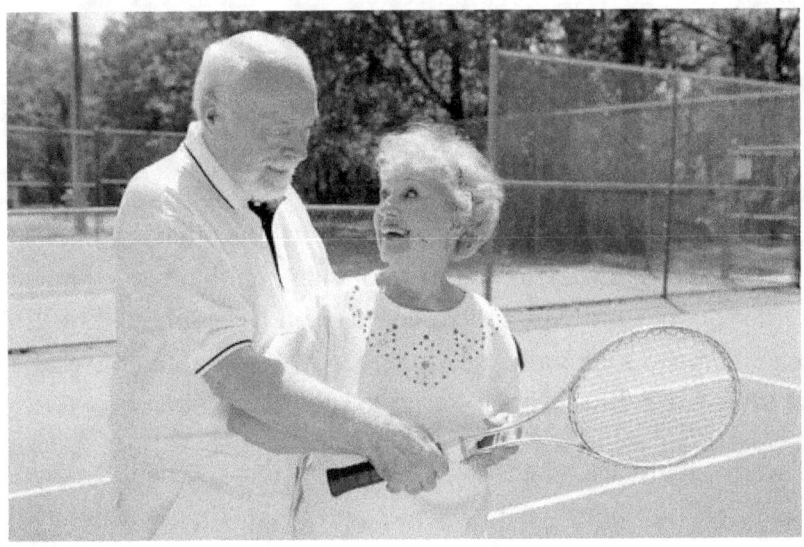

Around middle age, we start to notice the signs of aging: you get a gray hair that you can just pull out, your eyes start to have lines and wrinkles, and you might even make a noise when you get up. It is during this time that you start to notice that you are physically declining. Even those of us who are the most fit cannot get away unscathed. But you don't have to be like those who came before you!

My grandfather walks five miles every day. He eats what he wants, sleeps in, and sometimes enjoys a beer or two. However, he stays moving by cutting the grass, playing with his grandchildren, and taking dance lessons with my grandmother. Twice a week, he plays golf and walks instead of using the golf cart. He's 86 years old and still does everything for himself. He's old, and sometimes it is a little slower than it used to be, but he's still got it.

Aging isn't something we can outrun – a study done by the NIA found that people who ran marathons for over 20 years steadily added time to their records as they aged. They might have still been in great physical health, but they still took longer to complete the activity. Some physical decline is normal – you've put your body through a lot over its lifetime.

Many of these tips that you will read in this book come straight from gerontologists – or those who study what happens when we age. These scientists and doctors look for things that distinguish us as we age. They try to understand what health threats there are to older people and why older people seem to be targeted by diseases such as dementia or osteoporosis – and much of what that are finding links directly back to the body.

Of course there are other things that can affect our health as we age, things like family, stress, food, and even climate. But how we treat our bodies is a big part of that puzzle.

Gerontologists have been working with the National Institute on Aging and doing a study called the Baltimore Longitudinal Study of Aging, where they study these types of questions. They evaluate people over time to see how their bodies and minds react to different circumstances. The BLSA repeatedly evaluates people over time rather than comparing a group of young people to a group of old people, as in a cross-sectional study. Using this approach, BLSA scientists have observed, for example, that people who have no evidence of ear problems or noise-induced hearing loss still lose some of their hearing with age—that's normal. They use medical testing as well as informal testing – everything from simple puzzles like Sudoku to brain scans in a hospital.

What they found is that even people who stay healthy while they are aging still lose a lot of brain volume as they age – meaning that they lose the muscles in their cores, arms, abs, and legs – but also in their brains. This is important because even people who have the physical ability to work out or stay active lose the mental desire to go ahead and do it.

Whole Body Benefits for Exercise

As you age, exercise becomes more and more important to your body and mind. It's not really about adding years to your life, but giving you the ability to add life to your years.

Exercise helps you maintain or lose weight. You want to eat as you age, right? As we age, metabolism slows and maintaining a healthy weight is actually a lot harder. Exercise will help to increase that metabolism and build up your muscle mass – burning more calories. A healthy weight will keep you moving, but even more, it will allow you to eat just one more bite of pie without feeling guilty.

Exercise helps reduce the impact of chronic diseases and other illnesses. Among the many benefits of exercising, you will also have a better immune system, overall better hearth health, lower blood pressure, better bone density, and your digestion will improve. People who exercise also have a lowered risk of several chronic conditions including Alzheimer's disease, diabetes, obesity, heart disease, osteoporosis, and certain cancers.

Exercise enhances mobility, flexibility, and balance. With just one hour of exercise per day, you have improved strength, flexibility, and posture.

Better sleep quality. Poor sleep does not have to be a sign of gaining. Exercise will improve your sleep as you are tired enough to fall asleep quickly and sleep more deeply.

Better mood. There's a reason being a "grumpy old man" is a stereotype. Exercise will help to reduce endorphins, which will chase away some of those grumpy feelings. It also encourages you to be more self-confident – and who doesn't feel better when they have confidence?

Chapter 1: Starting Out

Starting out with an exercise routine is more important as you age than it ever was before. Regular exercise can and will boost your energy, help you stay independent, and manage your symptoms of illness and pain. Not only is exercise good for your body, but it is a way to keep you in high spirits and even help your memory. It doesn't matter if you are already feeling the pull of age or you are just trying to prevent it – we all have to start somewhere.

Exercise is your key to healthy aging.

You might feel discouraged before you even start exercising, whether you are plagued by health problems or not, but you need to start. If you've never really exercised before, it can be difficult to get into the swing of things. You might be afraid or think that you are too old or that exercise is not for you, but you would be wrong. Instead of thinking that you are "too" anything for exercise, you need to be honest.

Exercise and taking care of your body is the best way to age gracefully. It is really the way that you can stay energetic, stay strong, and stay healthy as you age – even if it sometimes makes you look not quite as good. Even more, it is a great way to stay connected with the world around you.

No matter what your current physical condition is or what you do, you can benefit from changing up your exercise routine in key ways. You won't have to run for hours on your treadmill or spend hours inside of a gym. Instead, it is more about adding movement into your daily life, even in small ways. You only have to work up to your own ability – you aren't in a competition here.

Even if you are housebound, there are ways to get it moving!

One of the biggest things that you need to overcome is your attitude – how can you properly get exercise if you aren't in the right mind frame? To combat that, we have a section of myths that we'd like to debunk:

Myth #1: I'm too old, there really isn't any point to exercise anyway.

Did you know that a 96 years old woman just ran a marathon? Exercising and strength training works to keep you feeling better and looking younger. Regular physical activity stops many forms of cancer, mind problems, and keeps your blood tests coming back at levels your doctor will appreciate. Not only will you see benefits, but you will feel benefits that you didn't even know you could feel.

Myth #2: Older generations shouldn't even exercise, instead they should rest and save their strength.

Actually, research shows that inactivity will lead you to declining at a faster rate. You will lose your strength and your speed. You will eventually lose the ability to even gain any of it back due to immobility, hospitalizations, or even medicines.

Myth #3: I will just fall down and hurt myself.

We all fall. However, regular exercise actually encourages your body to bounce back from injury and stops things like bone loss. As you exercise, you will see an improvement in balance, which will reduce your likelihood of falling.

Myth #4: I can't exercise sitting down.

If you cannot stand up or move your legs, you aren't forgotten here. Instead of walking or running, you can do things like lifting weights, stretching, chair aerobics and yoga, or even exercising in a pool. You will not only get a great core workout, but you will improve muscle tone and flexibility. Ask your doctor if there are any places where you can go that will help you with these exercises – many local colleges will offer them free of charge!

Tips for Getting Started with One Hour of Exercise a Day

Before you start working out, you will need to make a few different commitments to yourself that will keep you feeling and looking great.

Talk to your doctor. By talking for your doctor and getting a clearance for the exercise program, you will avoid any activities that could actually hurt you.

Consider health concerns. Look at your family history – are there any problems that your parents or grandparents faced? Make sure you do exercises that will help with those. Remember that certain exercises won't work for everyone, so make sure that you feel your body and understand what just doesn't feel right.

Start slow. If you haven't been active for a long time, it can be difficult to start and go all out with your routine. Instead, build up. While an hour is ideal, you can start at fifteen minutes and just f you just commit to making the move. After a few weeks, it will all become habit.

Set goals. Focus on setting short term goals that you will complete. Whether that is being able to walk a certain distance without stopping or working out five days a week, you are more likely to keep it up.

Recognize problems. If you hurt, stop exercising until someone can look at you. Stop exercising immediately and call your doctor if you feel dizzy or short of breath, develop chest pain or pressure, break out in a cold sweat, or experience pain. Also stop if a joint is red, swollen, or tender to touch.

Staying active and starting out is not anything that is rocket science. Instead, if it mixing together different kinds of exercise to keep you healthy and happy. The key is to find the activities that you enjoy and keeping your workouts interesting and fun.

Chapter 2: Cardio

There is no doubt in anyone's mind that cardio is probably the most important thing for staying and feeling young. Just one hour of cardio a day will keep your heart healthy and will have you moving again in no time. But one hour doesn't stop there. It will help your lungs, you liver, your muscles, and you brain.

If you can still move at all, no matter what the speed is, you are likely to be able to do some sort of cardio activity. Like we said before, if you can't get in an hour a day to start, never fear. You can build up to that. Intensity levels and activities can also vary.

To start shaping up your cardio, you need to decide what your favorite activity is. Examples of cardio include: walking, jogging, climbing stairs, hiking, and swimming.

You have to know your limits when you are doing your daily hour of cardio. If you have been inactive for a while, you can't start right away going in at an hour. Cardio tends to drain us of our strength faster, so you will need to really feel out your body.

If you aren't sure if you are working too much, you can do something called The Talk Test. If you can't get out enough words to make a sentence, you should sit back and take a break.

Form a Cardio Plan

When you go to do your cardio, pick an activity and see how it feels. If you don't like hiking, maybe swimming will be more up to your standards. You just need to make sure that whatever you do includes all three components of aerobic fitness: heart and lung performance, muscle endurance, and functional capacity.

Your daily hour of cardio should have three general parts:

High intensity exercise: You want to get your heart rate up as the best way to improve your lungs and heart. This will deliver blood and oxygen to your working muscles. High intensity is relative to each individual, so don't think you need to keep up with the 20 year old football player next to you. All you have to do to get your heart rate up to that level will depend on your current fitness level—it may be that a moderate walking pace up a small hill will work for you. As your fitness improves, you will likely have to work harder. Many people will figure out what their ideal heart rate is and then work from there.

> ➤ Plan to have three 20-minute sessions of high intensity cardio each week.

Moderate intensity: If you aren't feeling the high intensity exercises, then you can go for the moderate ones like bike riding or walking on flat ground. Playing tennis, volleyball, or golf (without a cart) will add the upper body work you need, as will swimming, water aerobics, and most other activities that involve continuous use of your upper and lower body muscles at the same time. You will build up endurance by doing this. The only downside is that you will need to fill your entire daily hour with this exercise, leaving little room for other types of sport.

Cool downs. Many people don't realize it, but cool downs are an integral part of your daily hour of exercise. The older you are, the more likely you are to have torn tendons, joints and the small muscles. If you do this, you won't be able to keep up your speed – especially because the older we are, the more time it takes for us to heal. Spend 5 minutes at the start of each exercise and 5 minutes at the end to stretch and slowly elevate and lower your heart rate.

To wrap it up:

Cardio uses large muscles groups and rhythmic motions over time to get your heart pumping and lungs working. You are likely to feel a little out of breath.

To get a cardio work out, include things into your exercise plan like walking, stair climbing, swimming, hiking, cycling, rowing, tennis, and dancing.

The result? You will have less fatigue when doing daily activities, less shortness of breath, and you will have more independence.

Chapter 3: Weight Training

Strength training doesn't just include "picking things up and putting them down," but rather it includes working and pushing your muscles in new, dynamic ways so that you keep your muscles guess.

Most doctors suggest that anyone over 50 does at least two days of weight training each and every week. It isn't as much the point to build your leg muscles so that they stick out or getting you a six pack, but it is for your overall health.

You can get a personalized plan from a personal trainer, or you can just do some of these at home techniques.

At home strength training:

Legs: Legs are one of the first things to fail on us, which is why it is important to keep them nice and strong. One of the best exercises is this one:

Sit erect in a chair with both of your feet firmly planted on the ground, keeping them shoulder width apart. Hold onto the sides of the chair if you don't feel steady, but you can also keep your arms straight in front of you. Start by lifting one leg off the floor until your knee is straight and parallel to the ground and hold that position for a few seconds. Then, return that leg to the starting position with both feet on the ground. Repeat on the other side. Work up to eight repetitions on each side – and then start doing eight, resting, doing eight more, and see how far you can go.

Arms: Your arms help you with everything from getting out of bed to lifting pots while you are cooking, so making sure that you keep them toned and worked is a great way to ensure that you can be independent. Here's a great exercise to do a few times a week:

Sit in a chair with your feet flat on the ground and your arms by your sides. Hold light weights in each hand – either weights that you would traditionally see or soup cans or water bottles if you don't have any. Hold your arms straight down by your sides with the palms facing inward. Keeping a small bend in your arm at the elbows, lift both arms out and up until they are perpendicular to your body or like you are making a cross. Hold for a count of three and then slowly go down. Pause and repeat 5-10 times. Do at least five sets – but build up if you can't.

Triceps Extensions

Another arm exercise is to start with your feet on the ground and one of your weights in your left hand. Bend that left elbow up straight to your ear so that it is pointing to the ceiling. You can use your right hand to support your left elbow so you don't hurt yourself. Slowly straighten your left arm to the ceiling. Hold this position for a count of three and then slowly lower back into the starting position. Do 5-10 times and then switch to your right side and repeat.

Abdominal Muscles: Your abdominal strength is key to your overall health. Your abs keep you sturdy and hardy as you do other exercises and go through your daily life. Exercises that work will include seated knee lifts, which you can do while sitting down.

Start by sitting with your feet on the ground and your back straight against the chair. Then, squeeze your abdominal muscles together and hold then while simultaneously raising your feet off the ground. Hold for a few seconds and release. Try to build up to six reps of this exercise and hold for a little longer over time.

Balance Exercises: Balance is key as we age, because a fall can be deadly. To keep your balance, you don't need to walk on a beam or a tightrope, but you can do little things. One of the best and easiest ways to up your balance is to walk heel-to-toe. You can use a wall or a cane for balance if need be. Walk slowly and carefully by playing the heel of your left foot directly in front of the toe of your right foot. Try to move quickly and continue walking in that way for at least six steps, but you can work it up so that you are doing many, many more!

To wrap it up:

You need strength training to build up your muscles. Work on things like weight or external resistance from body weight, machines, free weights, or elastic bands. Consider adding in power training, which combines moderate cardio and weight training for a better workout.

Strength training keeps your bones healthy, improves your balance, and builds up muscle. This will help so that you can avoid falls or at least to help you recover from them. Building strength and power will help you stay independent and make day-to-day activities easier such as opening a jar, getting in and out of a car, and lifting objects.

Chapter 4: Eating and Fitness

If you are getting in your hour of exercise each day, you should probably change up the way you eat. Not only will an hour a day of exercise keep you physically fit, but it will rev up your metabolism and have your body craving other types of foods.

For adults over 50 who are getting in an hour or more of fitness per day, eating a health benefit can only continue your quest for a fuller, healthier life. Healthy eating doesn't mean that you should chow down on chicken breasts and Brussels sprouts. After all, you are earning your scoop of ice cream or slice of cake.

Feed Your Mind, Body, and Soul

You probably have heard the old adage "You are what you eat." Remember that while it might not be exactly true, it is a good way to live. When you choose fruits that are vibrant, foods that are complex, and proteins that are lean, that is how you will look and feel.

Eating a meal that is balanced before you exercise, and refueling after you do your daily hour will leave you feeling stronger and living longer. Good nutrition keeps your muscles, bones, organs, and other body parts in the best condition. A proper diet reduces the risk of heart disease, stroke, high blood pressure, type-2 diabetes, bone loss, cancer, and anemia.

But it isn't all about your body – you want to sharpen your mind as well! People who eat a lot of brightly colored fruits and vegetables, leafy vegetables, fish and nuts packed with omega-3 fatty acids, and allow themselves to have sweets every now and again actually decrease their risk of Alzheimer's! Add in some antioxidant rich green tea to sip on instead of sodas and you will have better memory and mental alertness.

Most of all, eating better, you will feel better, and that is what it is all about.

How many calories do I need?

My grandfather always used to ask me, "Can you see a calorie?"

While the answer is no, there are some general rules you should follow.

A woman over 50 who spends 1 hour a day exercising needs 1800 calories a day to maintain her weight.

A man over 50 who spends 1 hour a day exercising needs 2200 calories a day to maintain his weight.

But still, eating 1800 calories a day of pure cake isn't going to get you anywhere.

Healthy eating as you age: Choosing healthy foods

Adults over fifty can feel better immediately if they try to change the way they eat. A balanced diet that is high in the following foods and an hour of physical activity each day contribute to a higher quality of life and enhanced independence as you age.

Fruits – focus on whole fruits instead of those juices. You want to get the fiber and vitamins that come from the entire thing. You should try to get 1-2 servings or more each day. Stop with the boring bananas and strawberries and instead go for berries and melons.

Vegetables – Color. Color. Color. Color is key when it comes to vegetables. Choose dark, leafy greens like kale and spinach for your salads and sandwiches. Add some carrots, squash or yams to your dinner plate. If you like to snack, try making kale chips with garlic or lemon.

Calcium – Bone health is critical as you work out so that you don't hurt yourself. Adults over 50 need 1,200 mg of calcium a day. You can get it through milk, yogurt, and cheese but you can also use non-dairy sources include tofu, broccoli, almonds, and kale.

Grains – Be smart with carbs, but don't try to avoid them. Avoidance means that you will just binge when you get the chance. Look for whole grain pasta, breads, and cereals. You will need 6-7 ounces a day, so keep it up – just try to avoid white flour.

Protein – When you are working out at any age, protein is key. Adults who are over 50 need about 1 to 1.5 grams per kilogram of bodyweight. This means that you will need anywhere from 68 to 102g of high quality protein if you weigh 150 pounds. Try to divide up your intake so that you feel fuller longer. Try to avoid getting most of your protein from red meat, and make sure to include fish, beans, peas, eggs, nuts, seeds, and low-fat milk and cheese in your diet.

Necessary Vitamins and Minerals

Water – Water is the most important drink in your house. As we age, we become more prone to dehydration, and that only goes up if we are doing an hour of exercise per day. Our bodies lose the ability to regulate fluid levels and we don't often feel as thirsty as we actually are. Try to get at least 64 fluid ounces of water in per day, and use a tracking app on your phone or just put a post it note up so that you remember. Sip every ten minutes or so to avoid urinary tract infections, constipation, and even confusion.

Always, always, always drink water with a meal as well to keep everything feeling great.

Vitamin B – As we age, our stomach starts to produce less and less gastric acid, which makes it hard for our bodies to absorb vitamin B-12, which is needed to keep our blood healthy and our nerves firing. Get the recommended daily intake (2.4 mcg) of B12 from fortified foods or a vitamin supplement and talk to your doctor about how to add more into your diet.

Vitamin D – Vitamin D is an essential part of our diets as it helps to keep calcium going so our bones are stronger and it helps with boosting muscles. We get most of it from our diets, which include fatty fish, egg yolks, and milks. However, we also get some vitamin D from the sun, so you might want to take your exercise outside if you can. However, with age comes extreme problems again, as our skin is less efficient at synthesizing vitamin D, so consult your doctor or dietician about supplementing your diet with fortified foods or a multivitamin, especially if you're obese or have limited sun exposure. And remember, it is so important to wear sunscreen.

Healthy eating as you age: Tips for wholesome eating

Once you've started to pay closer attention to your diet, you will start to notice when you have a "cheat" meal or you just don't feel right. But how can you get in that habit of eating well, especially if you've never really eaten that well before? Well there are a few keys that you can work on one at a time to improve your diet:

Step 1: Reduce Salt. Salt is a killer – it gives us high blood pressure and ups our fluid retention. Buy foods that a low in sodium and season your meals with things like garlic or herbs instead of salt.

Step 2: Enjoy healthy fats. Healthy fats are essential to your diet and your beauty. Try to add things like olive oil, avocados, salmon, walnuts, flaxseed, and other monounsaturated fats to your diet instead of unhealthy fats. These will work to help strengthen your heart and keep your bad LDL cholesterol levels low, while helping keep your good HDL levels high.

Step 3: Stop eating bad carbs. Avoid eating things like white flour, refined sugar, or white rice. All of these foods have been stripped of anything that is good for you. They digest quickly, but cause short lived energy followed by a bad crash. This means that you should pretty much avoid any packaged foods or things that are "quick." For long-lasting energy and stable insulin levels, choose "good" or complex carbs such as whole grains, beans, fruits, and vegetables.

Step 4: Cook, and cook smart. Cooking your own food is a great way to ensure that you are getting what you need. Prepare veggies by steaming or sautéing them in olive oil so that you get the most nutrients. Do not boil and do not fry, as these are basically ruining them.

Step 5: Get FIVE colors. The key to being healthy is colors, and you will know that you reached that peak when you have five colors on your plate. This is how the Japanese arrange their plates, and they are healthier and living longer than almost any other country in the world. Try to get five different colors on your plate, and jelly beans don't count!

Chapter 5: Create Your Fitness Plan

So saying that you will eat well and saying that you will get in your one hour of exercise per day is a great thing to say you will do, but can you actually do it without a plan? Probably not – people who plan out their fitness are more likely to stay on track.

Here is a SAMPLE plan that you can use to keep on your toes and stay physically active. This plan is just generic, and it in no way means that you have to do it this way. Your best bet is to talk to a doctor or a personal trainer to get something that will keep your physically fit and will work to your advantages. However, if you aren't in the position to pay for that type of treatment, this is a great place to start:

Monday:

Morning: Take a half hour walk around your neighborhood or at the local mall.

Afternoon: Work on some arm and leg strengthening activities for about 15-20 minutes.

Evening: Before going to bed, stretch out all of your muscles.

Tuesday:

Morning: 30 minutes of cycling at an incline of your choosing.

Afternoon: Work on some abs and core strengthening activities for about 15-20 minutes.

Evening: Before going to bed, stretch out all of your muscles.

Wednesday:

Morning: 30 minutes morning walk around your neighborhood, try to include some hills.

Afternoon: Work on some arm and leg strengthening activities for about 15-20 minutes.

Evening: Before going to bed, stretch out all of your muscles.

Thursday:

Morning: 30 minutes swim in your local pool – make sure that you are swimming and not floating!

Afternoon: Work on some abs and core strengthening activities for about 15-20 minutes.

Evening: Before going to bed, stretch out all of your muscles.

Friday:

Morning: 30 minute jog around your neighborhood.

Afternoon: Work on some arm and leg strengthening activities for about 15-20 minutes.

Evening: Before going to bed, stretch out all of your muscles.

Saturday

Morning: Take a hike with a group of friends.

Afternoon: Work on strengthening exercises for your weakest muscle group.

Evening: Before going to bed, stretch out all of your muscles.

Sunday:

Rest

Don't Forget

However, to make your plan work the best, you have to do one other thing: add more physical activity into your daily life. These won't count toward your daily hour, but they will extend it and make it easier!

Be active on the go – Skip over elevators and escalators and try to take the stairs. Park at the end of the parking lot instead of right at the front of the store. Walk down every aisle when grocery shopping. You can even practice some balance or strength exercises while doing any of the above – be creative!

Be active at home – Do some balancing exercises while watching your favorite television show. Try some wall pushups while you are waiting for your dinner to cook. Start walking to mow the lawn instead of riding. Rake leaves instead of using a blower. Start gardening. Play with your grandchildren. Do some leg lifts while on the phone with your verbose friend. Wherever you are or whatever you are doing, try to keep active!

Most importantly, however,

Be safe.

Nothing will stop you, unless you get an injury. This is when you have to use your common sense: don't exercise if you are ill or if something hurts very badly. Wear bright colors when you are walking on the roads. Don't exercise outdoors when it is slippery. Make sure you eat or drink a little something before you exercise.

Chapter 6: Home Gym Necessities

A lot of people, especially those who are a little older, like to work out at home, but it isn't always as effective as working out at a gym. However, if have a little extra money and the space, you can always set up your own workout zone in your house.

If you are going to build your home gym, you should at least utilize things like YouTube videos or on demand workout programs so that you can at least observe proper form. In order to get your own personal gym in your home, you need to at least have 10 essential items:

Dumbbells

Dumbbells are pretty much the essential items that you need in your own gym. They are easy to pick up at your local Target or Walmart and they are an immediate return on investment. Look for ones that are hex shaped that have a rubber coating. You should try to get 3-5 sets, starting with a light pair, a normal pair, and an aspirational point.

Kettlebell

Many people will try to tell you that a kettlebell isn't something that you definitely need, but it really is. The movements that you can do with a kettlebell are similar to those you can do with a dumbbell, but you can do many of them standing up because you have balance. Certain of the movements that you can do are unique, and are particularly good for your hip flexors. Look for the kettlebells that have smooth handles but do not have a painted coating.

Pull Up Bar

Pull up bars might confuse you, especially if you don't have a lot of strength, but they aren't just to pull ups! You can do a lot of basic gymnastic exercises and strength exercises with this – and you can ever try some pull ups. Most pull up bars are built for doorways, so you should have someone install it that knows what they are doing. Make sure you pay attention to the weight requirements, because a fall could be devastating.

Rings

This is a great option for home or travel because they are super lightweight and great for bodyweight exercises. Rings will give you the ability to add a whole variety of weight exercises that also improve your flexibility and body strength. You will have to hang these as well, so make sure that you do it well before you hurt yourself.

Jump Rope

Just like the ones that you had in elementary school, jump ropes are actually much more of a workout than you think it is. It is harder than you remember, but it is also great for leg strength and cardio. Plus, you work on your coordination. Get a rope that is durable and strong. If you want to work on speed, go for lightweight ropes. If you want to go for strength, you can get weighted ropes.

Medicine Ball

Plyometric exercise is easy with a medicine ball, plus it makes exercise a lot more fun. You can work on muscles, cardio, and your core with a medicine ball by throwing, carrying, or doing exercises on it. This one is one of the most flexible tools you will have in your gym! Look for one that is soft, meaning that it is forgiving, so that it is easier to catch or rest on. Err on the lighter side when it comes to your medicine ball purchases as you want to focus on speed and power here, not so much strength.

Plyo Box

If there is something on this list that you don't know about, it is the Plyo Box. This will help you with stepping up, squatting, resting, bench dips, and other jumping and non-jumping exercises. You can build your own so that you can be super specific with it, or you can go to the store and get your own. There is also a great selection online!

Barbell

No gym, home or otherwise, would be complete without a barbell. These are also free weights and are so much better than the machines that you see at the gym because they allow for more dynamic actions. You will not only work on strength, but also on stabilization and coordination. Look for a barbell that is sturdy, but you don't have to break the bank on this. Pay attention to things like the diameter. If you don't have a lot of strength, consider purchasing a woman's bar, which tends to be thinner and lighter.

Weight Plates

A bar without anything on it is just silly! Buy a variety of plates that will let you do different exercises, including – 2.5#, 5#, 10#, 25# and, if you are fairly strong, 45# plates. You might also want to invest in some mats to make your workout safer.

Radio

While this might seem a little silly, having a radio will definitely help you out. Plus, if you have a radio or better yet, a television, you will be able to follow different exercise programs.

With these ten items and a little bit of decoration, you could have yourself a great gym. There are tons of other things you could add: yoga mats, yoga balls, stationary bikes, water cooler, and even mirrors.

Most importantly, make sure that you have some sort of safety set up. Whether you wear a Life Alert badge or you only exercise when someone is home, it is important to have access to proper medical care or have someone who can make the phone call.

Conclusion

At the end of the day, an hour of exercise a day isn't really a big commitment, but it can make a really big change to your life. You are more than your body, but your body is the vessel that will help you stay involved in your grandchildren's lives, your children's lives, and it will even help keep you a participating member of society.

The more you exercise, the more you will reap the benefits of each and every workout. Remember to space things out and try your hardest to push yourself, but stay within your limits. It is especially important to start out by working with your doctor or a trainer so that you can understand what your limits are and what your goals should be.

Now that you've started, however, if you ever stop, you are going to feel it. So you should know that there are ways to stay inspired about your fitness journey:

Keep a log

Keeping a log is a great way to see your daily hour (or more) that will have you feeling and looking much younger than you are.

Stay inspired about your transformation

While you will see results, they might not happen right away. Keep yourself moving by staying inspired by watching sports shows or reading magazines – soon you could be in one of them!

Get support from friends and family.

Everyone can benefit from having a little more activity in their lives, so bring someone with you. You could also sign up for a class that will have people similar to you working out.

No matter what, this hour is going to change you. One hour out of the day that is all about you is pretty much one of the best things you can do for yourself. Keep it up!

We will end with a quote that I hope you find inspiration:

If you always put limits on everything you do, physical or anything else, it will spread into your work and into your life. There are no limits. There are only plateaus; and you must not stay there, you must go beyond them."
-- Bruce Lee

Take away those limits and go be the best possible you that you can be.

Check Out Other Books

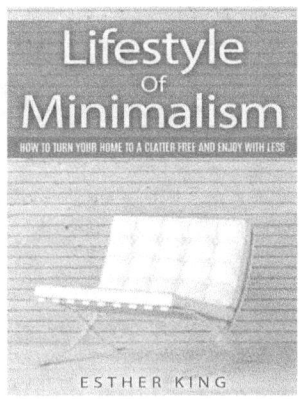

Lifestyle Of Minimalism: How To Turn Your Home to a Clutter Free and Enjoy With Less.

http://www.amazon.com/Lifestyle-Minimalism-Turn-Clutter-Enjoy-ebook/dp/B00WYSZRFY

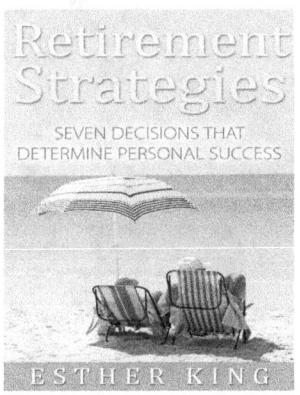

Retirement Strategies: Seven Decisions that Determine Personal Success.

http://www.amazon.com/Retirement-Strategies-Decisions-Determine-Personal-ebook/dp/B00ZNODHA8

www.ingramcontent.com/pod-product-compliance
Lightning Source LLC
Chambersburg PA
CBHW062030280526
45787CB00005B/2275